OSTEOPOROSIS JUICING AND SMOOTHIES FOR SENIORS OVER 50

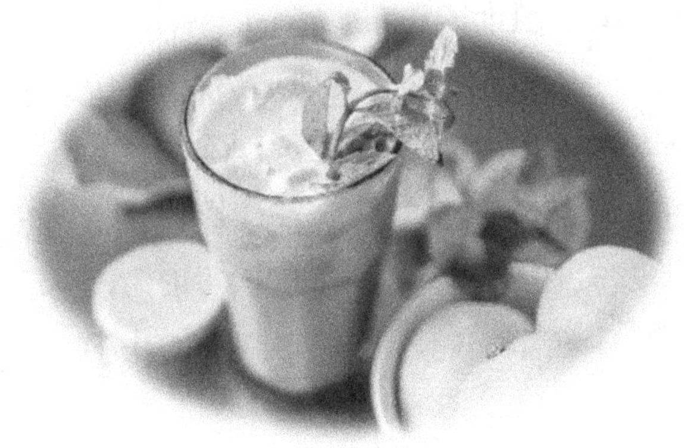

Nutritious blends for healthy and strong bones

Dr. Fawn Henry

Copyright © [2024] by [Dr. Fawn Henry]

Reserved all rights. This publication cannot be duplicated, shared, or transmitted in any way without the publisher's prior written consent. The only exceptions are brief quotes used in critical evaluations and certain other noncommercial uses allowed by copyright law. Such uses include photocopying, recording, and other electronic or mechanical methods

INTRODUCTION

Welcome to the "Juicing and Smoothies Osteoporosis Cookbook for Seniors Over 50: Delicious and Nutritious Low-Carb and Low-Sugar Recipes for Elders." I'm thrilled to embark on this journey with you as we delve into the transformative power of nutrition in managing osteoporosis and enhancing overall health.

As a seasoned nutritionist with years of experience, I've witnessed firsthand the profound impact that diet can have on our well-being. My passion for nutrition stems from a deeply personal experience—a journey that began with a dear friend named Sarah.

Sarah was not just a friend; she was family—a vibrant soul whose zest for life was unparalleled. However, her joyous spirit was overshadowed by the debilitating effects of osteoporosis. The relentless pain, the fear of fractures, and the limitations imposed by this condition threatened to dim her radiant light.

Determined to help Sarah reclaim her vitality, I embarked on a mission to explore the intersection of nutrition and osteoporosis management. What I discovered was nothing short of remarkable. Through a tailored regimen of nutrient-dense juices and smoothies, Sarah experienced a remarkable transformation. Her pain diminished, her bone density improved, and her once-diminished hope was reignited.

Sarah's journey serves as a testament to the incredible potential of food as medicine. It was not just about nourishing her body; it was about empowering her to take control of her health and embrace life with renewed vigor. Inspired by Sarah's resilience and the countless individuals facing similar challenges, I set out to create this cookbook—a beacon of hope for those navigating the complexities of osteoporosis.

Within these pages, you'll discover a treasure trove of delicious and nutritious recipes meticulously crafted to support bone health, reduce inflammation, and tantalize your taste buds. Each recipe is thoughtfully curated to be low in carbohydrates and sugar, aligning with the dietary needs of seniors over 50 managing osteoporosis.

But this cookbook is more than just a collection of recipes; it's a comprehensive guide to holistic wellness. You'll find invaluable insights into the science behind osteoporosis, practical tips for incorporating juicing and smoothies into your daily routine, and empowering strategies for enhancing your overall health and vitality.

Whether you're seeking relief from the symptoms of osteoporosis, striving to prevent its onset, or simply looking to optimize your well-being, this cookbook is your trusted companion on the path to vibrant health.

Join me as we embark on a journey of nourishment, healing, and empowerment. Together, let's unlock the transformative power of nutrition and embrace a life of vitality, one delicious sip at a time.

CHAPTER 1

Osteoporosis:

Osteoporosis is a prevalent but often underestimated condition characterized by weakened bones, making them fragile and susceptible to fractures. Derived from the Greek words "osteo," meaning bone, and "porosis," meaning porous, osteoporosis literally translates to "porous bone." While it's commonly associated with aging, osteoporosis can affect individuals of all ages and genders, although it disproportionately impacts older adults, particularly postmenopausal women.

Types of Osteoporosis:

1. **Primary Osteoporosis**: This is the most common type of osteoporosis and typically occurs due to the natural aging process. Primary osteoporosis is further divided into two subtypes:

   - **Postmenopausal Osteoporosis:** Occurs in women after menopause due to decreased estrogen levels, which accelerates bone loss.

- Age-Related Osteoporosis: Affects both men and women as they age, leading to gradual loss of bone density.

2. **Secondary Osteoporosis**: This type of osteoporosis develops as a result of underlying medical conditions or medications that adversely affect bone health. Examples include hormonal disorders, gastrointestinal diseases, prolonged corticosteroid use, and certain cancer treatments.

Causes of Osteoporosis:

Understanding the underlying causes of osteoporosis is crucial for effective prevention and management. Several factors contribute to the development of this condition:

1. **Hormonal Changes:** Hormones play a significant role in maintaining bone density. Reduced estrogen levels in postmenopausal women and low testosterone levels in men can accelerate bone loss and increase the risk of osteoporosis.

2. **Nutritional Deficiencies**: Inadequate intake of calcium, vitamin D, and other essential nutrients essential for bone health can impair bone formation and weaken bone structure.

3. **Sedentary Lifestyle**: Lack of weight-bearing exercise and physical activity can lead to decreased bone density and strength.

4. **Genetics:** Family history and genetic predisposition can influence an individual's susceptibility to osteoporosis.

5. **Medications:** Certain medications, such as long-term corticosteroids, anticonvulsants, and proton pump inhibitors, can interfere with bone metabolism and increase the risk of osteoporosis.

Symptoms of Osteoporosis:

Osteoporosis is often referred to as the "silent disease" because it typically progresses without noticeable symptoms until a fracture occurs. However, there are some signs and symptoms to be aware of:

1. **Back Pain**: Persistent or sudden onset of back pain, caused by vertebral fractures or collapsed vertebrae, is a common symptom of osteoporosis.

2. **Loss of Height**: As osteoporosis progresses, individuals may experience a gradual loss of height due to compression fractures in the spine.

3. **Fractures:** Osteoporosis-related fractures can occur in various bones, including the spine, hip, wrist, and ribs. Fractures may occur spontaneously or as a result of minimal trauma.

Preventive Measures for Osteoporosis:

While certain risk factors for osteoporosis, such as age and genetics, are beyond our control, there are proactive steps individuals can take to reduce their risk and promote bone health:

1. **Maintain a Balanced Diet**: Consume a diet rich in calcium, vitamin D, magnesium, and other nutrients essential for bone health. Good dietary sources of calcium include dairy products, leafy green vegetables, and fortified foods. Adequate vitamin D can be obtained from sunlight exposure and supplementation if necessary.

2. **Engage in Weight-Bearing Exercise**: Regular weight-bearing exercise, such as walking, jogging, dancing, and resistance training, helps stimulate bone formation and increase bone density.

3. **Avoid Smoking and Excessive Alcohol Consumption:** Smoking and excessive alcohol intake have been linked to accelerated bone loss and increased fracture risk. Quitting smoking and limiting alcohol consumption can help preserve bone health.

4. **Get Regular Bone Density Screenings**: Bone density testing, such as dual-energy X-ray absorptiometry (DXA) scans, can assess bone density and identify individuals at risk of osteoporosis or osteopenia.

5. **Discuss Medication Risks with Your Healthcare Provider:** If you're taking medications known to affect bone health, such as corticosteroids or anticonvulsants, discuss potential risks with your healthcare provider and explore alternative treatment options if necessary.

6. **Fall Prevention**: Take measures to reduce the risk of falls, such as removing tripping hazards from your home, installing handrails and grab bars, and wearing supportive footwear.

CHAPTER 2

In crafting a juicing and smoothie guide for seniors over 50 managing osteoporosis, it's essential to highlight not just what to include but also what to avoid to ensure optimal bone health and overall well-being. Here are some key points to consider when selecting ingredients for your recipes:

1. **High-Sugar Fruits and Sweeteners**: While fruits can add natural sweetness and flavor to juices and smoothies, it's important to choose low-sugar options to prevent blood sugar spikes and promote stable energy levels. Avoid using fruits with high glycemic index values, such as bananas, mangoes, and pineapples, in excess. Instead, opt for berries, apples, pears, and citrus fruits, which are lower in sugar and rich in vitamins, antioxidants, and fiber.

2. **Excessive Oxalate-Rich Greens**: Leafy greens like spinach, Swiss chard, and beet greens are nutritious additions to juices and smoothies, providing essential vitamins and minerals.

However, these greens are also high in oxalates, compounds that can interfere with calcium absorption and contribute to the formation of kidney stones. While moderate consumption of oxalate-rich greens is generally safe for most individuals, seniors with a history of kidney stones or calcium oxalate issues may benefit from limiting their intake.

3. **Caffeinated and Sugary Beverages**: Juices and smoothies should serve as nourishing beverages that support bone health, rather than sources of empty calories and stimulants. Avoid adding caffeinated beverages like coffee and energy drinks, as well as sugary fruit juices and sweetened dairy products, which can contribute to inflammation and negatively impact calcium balance. Instead, focus on hydrating with water, herbal teas, or unsweetened plant-based milks like almond or coconut milk.

4. **Excessive Sodium and Processed Ingredients:**
   Processed foods and condiments high in sodium can disrupt calcium metabolism and contribute to bone loss over time. When preparing juices and smoothies, steer clear of processed ingredients like canned fruits, vegetable juices with added salt, and packaged smoothie mixes containing artificial flavors and preservatives. Instead, prioritize whole, minimally processed ingredients like fresh fruits, vegetables, nuts, seeds, and herbs to maximize nutrient intake and support bone health.

5. **Acidic Ingredients:** Acidic foods can increase the acidity of the body's pH levels, leading to calcium leaching from the bones in an attempt to buffer the acid load. While some acidity is normal and necessary for proper digestion and metabolism, excessive consumption of acidic foods may exacerbate bone loss and weaken bone density. Limit acidic ingredients like citrus fruits, tomatoes, vinegar, and spicy peppers in your juices and smoothies, and balance them with alkalizing ingredients like leafy greens, cucumbers, and celery to maintain optimal pH balance.

By being mindful of these considerations and avoiding potentially detrimental ingredients, seniors over 50 can create delicious and nutritious juices and smoothies that support bone health, reduce inflammation, and enhance overall well-being. Remember to focus on variety, moderation, and balance in your recipes to achieve optimum health and vitality at any age.

CHAPTER 3

breakfast recipes:

1. **Avocado and Egg Breakfast Salad**

Ingredients:

- 1 ripe avocado, diced
- 2 hard-boiled eggs, sliced
- 1 cup cherry tomatoes, halved
- 2 cups baby spinach
- 1 tablespoon extra virgin olive oil
- 1 tablespoon lemon juice
- Salt and pepper to taste

Instructions:

8. In a large bowl, combine avocado, eggs, cherry tomatoes, and baby spinach.

9. Drizzle with olive oil and lemon juice.

10. Season with salt and pepper to taste.

11. Gently toss to coat.

12. Serve immediately.

Servings: 2 **Nutritional Value per serving:** Calories: 280 | Protein: 10g | Carbohydrates: 14g | Fat: 21g | Fiber: 9g **Preparation Time:** 10 minutes

2. Greek Yogurt Parfait

Ingredients:

- 1 cup plain Greek yogurt

- 1/2 cup mixed berries (strawberries, blueberries, raspberries)

- 2 tablespoons chopped almonds

- 1 tablespoon honey (optional)

Instructions:

4. In a serving glass or bowl, layer Greek yogurt, mixed berries, and chopped almonds.

5. Drizzle with honey if desired.

6. Repeat layers until ingredients are used up.

7. Serve chilled.

Servings: 1 **Nutritional Value per serving:** Calories: 300 | Protein: 20g | Carbohydrates: 25g | Fat: 15g | Fiber: 5g
Preparation Time: 5 minutes

3. **Spinach and Mushroom Omelette**

Ingredients:

- 2 large eggs

- 1 cup fresh spinach leaves

- 1/2 cup sliced mushrooms

- 1/4 cup diced onions

- 1 tablespoon olive oil

- Salt and pepper to taste

Instructions:

6. In a bowl, whisk eggs until well beaten.

7. Heat olive oil in a non-stick skillet over medium heat.

8. Add onions and mushrooms, sauté until softened.

9. Add spinach leaves and cook until wilted.

10. Pour beaten eggs over the vegetables in the skillet.

11. Cook until eggs are set, then fold the omelette in half.

12. Season with salt and pepper to taste.

13. Serve hot.

Servings: 1 **Nutritional Value per serving:** Calories: 250 | Protein: 15g | Carbohydrates: 7g | Fat: 18g | Fiber: 3g **Preparation Time:** 15 minutes

4. Chia Seed Pudding

Ingredients:

- 2 tablespoons chia seeds

- 1/2 cup unsweetened almond milk

- 1/4 teaspoon vanilla extract

- 1 tablespoon honey or maple syrup (optional)

- Fresh fruit for topping (e.g., berries, sliced banana)

Instructions:

5. In a bowl, combine chia seeds, almond milk, vanilla extract, and sweetener if using.

6. Stir well to combine.

7. Let the mixture sit for 5 minutes, then stir again to prevent clumping.

8. Cover and refrigerate for at least 2 hours or overnight until thickened.

9. Serve topped with fresh fruit.

Servings: 1 **Nutritional Value per serving:** Calories: 180 | Protein: 5g | Carbohydrates: 20g | Fat: 9g | Fiber: 10g
Preparation Time: 5 minutes (+ chilling time)

5. Quinoa Breakfast Bowl

Ingredients:

- 1/2 cup cooked quinoa

- 1/4 cup Greek yogurt

- 1/4 cup mixed berries

- 1 tablespoon chopped nuts (e.g., almonds, walnuts)

- 1 teaspoon honey or maple syrup (optional)

- Cinnamon for sprinkling

Instructions:

6. In a bowl, layer cooked quinoa, Greek yogurt, mixed berries, and chopped nuts.

7. Drizzle with honey or maple syrup if desired.

8. Sprinkle with cinnamon.

9. Serve immediately.

Servings: 1 Nutritional Value per serving: Calories: 280 | Protein: 12g | Carbohydrates: 40g | Fat: 8g | Fiber: 6g **Preparation Time:** 10 minutes

6. **Smoked Salmon and Avocado Toast**

Ingredients:

- 2 slices whole grain bread, toasted

- 1/2 ripe avocado, mashed

- 2 ounces smoked salmon

- 1 tablespoon capers

- Fresh dill for garnish

- Lemon wedges for serving

Instructions:

6. Spread mashed avocado evenly on toasted bread slices.

7. Top each slice with smoked salmon and capers.

8. Garnish with fresh dill.

9. Serve with lemon wedges on the side.

Servings: 1 **Nutritional Value per serving:** Calories: 320 | Protein: 20g | Carbohydrates: 25g | Fat: 15g | Fiber: 8g **Preparation Time:** 10 minutes

7. **Sweet Potato Breakfast Hash**

Ingredients:

- 1 small sweet potato, peeled and diced

- 1/4 cup diced bell peppers

- 1/4 cup diced onions

- 2 eggs

- 1 tablespoon olive oil

- Salt and pepper to taste

- Fresh parsley for garnish

Instructions:

7. Heat olive oil in a skillet over medium heat.

8. Add diced sweet potato, bell peppers, and onions to the skillet.

9. Cook until sweet potato is tender and lightly browned.

10. Make two wells in the hash and crack an egg into each well.

11. Cook until eggs are set to your desired doneness.

12. Season with salt and pepper to taste.

13. Garnish with fresh parsley.

14. Serve hot.

Servings: 1 **Nutritional Value per serving:** Calories: 350 | Protein: 14g | Carbohydrates: 30g | Fat: 18g | Fiber: 5g **Preparation Time:** 20 minutes

8. **Cottage Cheese and Fruit Bowl**

Ingredients:

- 1/2 cup low-fat cottage cheese

- 1/2 cup mixed berries

- 1 tablespoon chopped nuts (e.g., almonds, walnuts)

- 1 teaspoon honey or maple syrup (optional)

- Cinnamon for sprinkling

Instructions:

5. berries, and chopped nuts.

6. In a bowl, layer cottage cheese, mixed Drizzle with honey or maple syrup if desired.

7. Sprinkle with cinnamon.

8. Serve immediately.

Servings: 1 **Nutritional Value per serving:** Calories: 250 | Protein: 20g | Carbohydrates: 20g | Fat: 10g | Fiber: 5g

Preparation Time: 5 minutes

9. Green Smoothie Bowl

Ingredients:

- 1 cup baby spinach

- 1/2 ripe avocado

- 1/2 cup frozen mixed berries

- 1/2 cup unsweetened almond milk

- 1 tablespoon chia seeds

- 1 tablespoon honey or maple syrup (optional)

- Toppings: sliced banana, granola, chopped nuts

Instructions:

7. In a blender, combine baby spinach, avocado, frozen mixed berries, almond milk, chia seeds, and sweetener if using.

8. Blend until smooth and creamy.

9. Pour the smoothie into a bowl.

10. Top with sliced banana, granola, and chopped nuts.

11. Serve immediately.

Servings: 1 **Nutritional Value per serving:** Calories: 350 | Protein: 10g | Carbohydrates: 40g | Fat: 18g | Fiber: 12g **Preparation Time:** 5 minutes

10. Egg and Veggie Breakfast Wrap

Ingredients:
- 2 large eggs, beaten
- 1 whole grain or gluten-free wrap
- 1/4 cup chopped bell peppers
- 1/4 cup chopped onions
- 1/4 cup diced tomatoes
- 1/4 cup shredded low-fat cheese
- 1 tablespoon olive oil
- Salt and pepper to taste

Instructions:
1. Heat olive oil in a skillet over medium heat.
2. Add chopped bell peppers, onions, and tomatoes to the skillet.
3. Sauté until vegetables are tender.
4. Pour beaten eggs into the skillet and cook until scrambled.
5. Season with salt and pepper to taste.
6. Place the cooked egg mixture in the center of the wrap.
7. Top with shredded cheese.
8. Roll up the wrap and serve.

Servings: 1 **Nutritional Value per serving:** Calories: 350 | Protein: 20g | Carbohydrates: 25g | Fat: 18g | Fiber: 5g
Preparation Time: 15 minutes

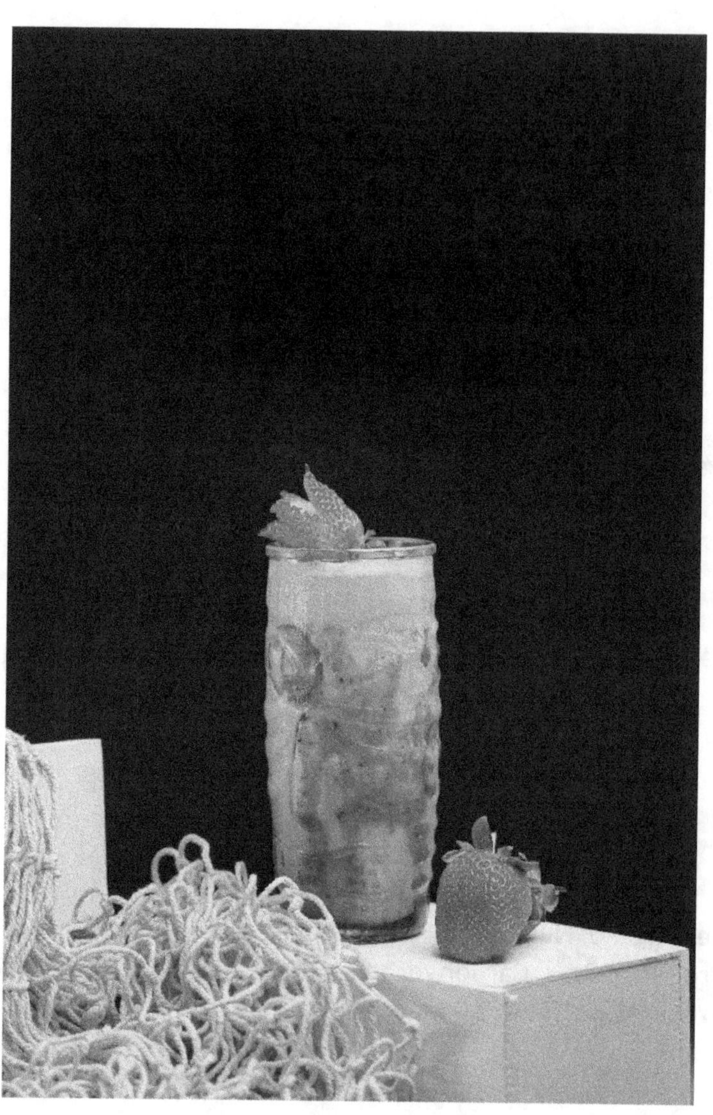

CHAPTER 4

LUNCH RECIPES:

2. **Grilled Salmon Salad**

Ingredients:

- 2 salmon fillets

- 4 cups mixed greens

- 1/2 cup cherry tomatoes, halved

- 1/4 cup cucumber, sliced

- 1/4 cup red onion, thinly sliced

- 2 tablespoons olive oil

- 1 tablespoon lemon juice

- Salt and pepper to taste

Instructions:

9. Preheat grill to medium-high heat.

10. Season salmon fillets with salt, pepper, and a drizzle of olive oil.

11. Grill salmon for 4-5 minutes on each side, or until cooked through.

12. In a large bowl, toss mixed greens, cherry tomatoes, cucumber, and red onion with olive oil and lemon juice.

13. Divide salad mixture onto plates and top with grilled salmon fillets.

14. Serve immediately.

Servings: 2 **Nutritional Value per serving:** Calories: 350 | Protein: 30g | Carbohydrates: 10g | Fat: 20g | Fiber: 4g **Preparation Time:** 20 minutes

2. Quinoa Stuffed Bell Peppers

Ingredients:

- 2 large bell peppers, halved and seeds removed

- 1 cup cooked quinoa

- 1/2 cup black beans, drained and rinsed

- 1/2 cup diced tomatoes

- 1/4 cup diced red onion

- 1/4 cup shredded low-fat cheese

- 1 tablespoon olive oil

- 1 teaspoon chili powder

- Salt and pepper to taste

Instructions:

9. Preheat oven to 375°F (190°C).

10. In a bowl, combine cooked quinoa, black beans, diced tomatoes, red onion, shredded cheese, olive oil, chili powder, salt, and pepper.

11. Fill each bell pepper half with the quinoa mixture.

12. Place stuffed bell peppers on a baking sheet lined with parchment paper.

13. Bake for 25-30 minutes, or until bell peppers are tender and filling is heated through.

14. Serve hot.

Servings: 2 **Nutritional Value per serving:** Calories: 300 | Protein: 12g | Carbohydrates: 35g | Fat: 12g | Fiber: 8g **Preparation Time:** 40 minutes

3. **Turkey and Avocado Wrap**

Ingredients:

- 2 whole grain or gluten-free wraps

- 4 ounces sliced turkey breast

- 1/2 avocado, sliced

- 1/4 cup shredded lettuce

- 2 tablespoons hummus

- 1 tablespoon Dijon mustard

- Salt and pepper to taste

Instructions:

7. Lay out wraps on a clean surface.

8. Spread hummus evenly on each wrap, leaving a border around the edges.

9. Layer sliced turkey, avocado, and shredded lettuce on top of the hummus.

10. Drizzle with Dijon mustard and season with salt and pepper.

11. Roll up wraps tightly and slice in half.

12. Serve immediately or wrap in foil for later.

Servings: 2 **Nutritional Value per serving:** Calories: 320 |
Protein: 20g | Carbohydrates: 30g | Fat: 15g | Fiber: 8g
Preparation Time: 10 minutes

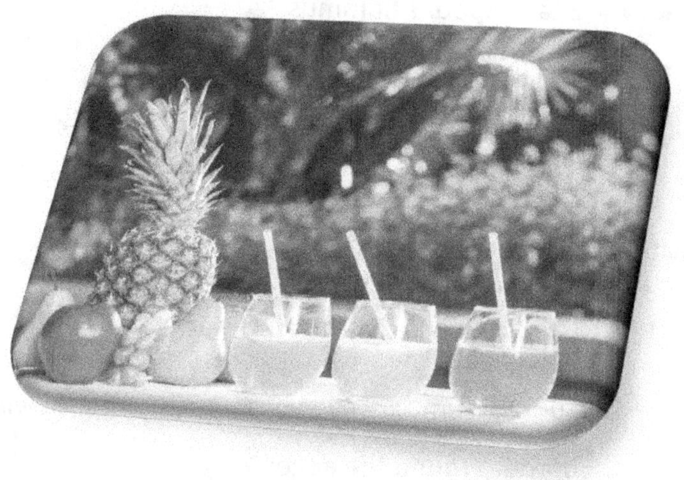

4. **Mediterranean Chickpea Salad**

Ingredients:

- 1 can (15 ounces) chickpeas, drained and rinsed

- 1 cup cucumber, diced

- 1 cup cherry tomatoes, halved

- 1/4 cup red onion, thinly sliced

- 1/4 cup Kalamata olives, pitted and sliced

- 2 tablespoons crumbled feta cheese

- 2 tablespoons olive oil

- 1 tablespoon lemon juice

- 1 teaspoon dried oregano

- Salt and pepper to taste

Instructions:

10. In a large bowl, combine chickpeas, cucumber, cherry tomatoes, red onion, Kalamata olives, and feta cheese.

11. Drizzle olive oil and lemon juice over the salad.

12. Sprinkle with dried oregano, salt, and pepper.

13. Toss gently to combine.

14. Serve chilled or at room temperature.

Servings: 2 **Nutritional Value per serving:** Calories: 320 |
Protein: 12g | Carbohydrates: 35g | Fat: 15g | Fiber: 10g
Preparation Time: 15 minutes

5. **Eggplant and Zucchini Ratatouille**

Ingredients:

- 1 eggplant, diced

- 2 zucchinis, diced

- 1 bell pepper, diced

- 1 onion, diced

- 2 cloves garlic, minced

- 1 can (15 ounces) diced tomatoes

- 1 tablespoon olive oil

- 1 teaspoon dried thyme

- 1 teaspoon dried basil

- Salt and pepper to taste

Instructions:

10. Heat olive oil in a large skillet over medium heat.

11. Add diced eggplant, zucchini, bell pepper, onion, and garlic to the skillet.

12. Cook until vegetables are softened, about 10 minutes.

13. Stir in diced tomatoes, dried thyme, dried basil, salt, and pepper.

14. Simmer for an additional 10 minutes, stirring occasionally.

15. Serve hot, garnished with fresh herbs if desired.

Servings: 4 **Nutritional Value per serving:** Calories: 150 | Protein: 3g | Carbohydrates: 20g | Fat: 7g | Fiber: 8g **Preparation Time:** 30 minutes

6. **Lentil and Vegetable Soup**

Ingredients:

- 1 cup dried green lentils, rinsed

- 4 cups vegetable broth

- 1 onion, diced

- 2 carrots, diced

- 2 celery stalks, diced

- 2 cloves garlic, minced

- 1 teaspoon dried thyme

- 1 teaspoon dried rosemary

- Salt and pepper to taste

Instructions:

9. In a large pot, combine dried lentils, vegetable broth, diced onion, carrots, celery, garlic, dried thyme, dried rosemary, salt, and pepper.

10. Bring to a boil, then reduce heat to low and simmer for 20-25 minutes, or until lentils are tender.

11. Taste and adjust seasoning if necessary.

12. Serve hot, garnished with fresh herbs if desired.

Servings: 4 **Nutritional Value per serving:** Calories: 200 | Protein: 12g | Carbohydrates: 35g | Fat: 1g | Fiber: 12g **Preparation Time:** 30 minutes

7. **Tuna Salad Lettuce Wraps**

Ingredients:

- 1 can (5 ounces) tuna, drained

- 1/4 cup diced celery

- 2 tablespoons diced red onion

- 2 tablespoons plain Greek yogurt

- 1 tablespoon lemon juice

- 1 teaspoon Dijon mustard

- Salt and pepper to taste

- Butter lettuce leaves for wrapping

Instructions:

8. In a bowl, combine drained tuna, diced celery, diced red onion, Greek yogurt, lemon juice, Dijon mustard, salt, and pepper.

9. Mix until well combined.

10. Spoon tuna salad onto butter lettuce leaves.

11. Roll up lettuce leaves to form wraps.

12. Serve immediately.

Servings: 2 **Nutritional Value per serving:** Calories: 150 |
Protein: 20g | Carbohydrates: 5g | Fat: 5g | Fiber: 2g
Preparation Time: 10 minutes

8. **Broccoli and Cauliflower Salad**

Ingredients:

- 2 cups broccoli florets

- 2 cups cauliflower florets

- 1/4 cup diced red onion

- 1/4 cup sunflower seeds

- 2 tablespoons dried cranberries

- 2 tablespoons plain Greek yogurt

- 1 tablespoon apple cider vinegar

- 1 teaspoon honey (optional)

- Salt and pepper to taste

Instructions:

9. Steam broccoli and cauliflower florets until tender, then rinse under cold water to cool.

10. In a large bowl, combine steamed broccoli and cauliflower with diced red onion, sunflower seeds, and dried cranberries.

11. In a small bowl, whisk together Greek yogurt, apple cider vinegar, honey (if using), salt, and pepper.

12. Pour dressing over the salad and toss to coat evenly.

13. Serve chilled or at room temperature.

Servings: 2 **Nutritional Value per serving:** Calories: 180 | Protein: 8g | Carbohydrates: 20g | Fat: 8g | Fiber: 6g **Preparation Time:** 15 minutes

9. **Veggie and Hummus Wrap**

Ingredients:

- 2 whole grain or gluten-free wraps

- 1/4 cup hummus

- 1/2 cup shredded lettuce

- 1/2 cup shredded carrots

- 1/2 cup sliced cucumber

- 1/4 cup sliced bell peppers

- Salt and pepper to taste

Instructions:

7. Lay out wraps on a clean surface.

8. Spread hummus evenly on each wrap, leaving a border around the edges.

9. Layer shredded lettuce, shredded carrots, sliced cucumber, and sliced bell peppers on top of the hummus.

10. Season with salt and pepper.

11. Roll up wraps tightly and slice in half.

12. Serve immediately or wrap in foil for later.

Servings: 2 **Nutritional Value per serving:** Calories: 200 | Protein: 6g | Carbohydrates: 25g | Fat: 8g | Fiber: 6g **Preparation Time:** 10 minutes

10. Black Bean and Corn Salad

Ingredients:

- 1 can (15 ounces) black beans, drained and rinsed

- 1 cup frozen corn kernels, thawed

- 1/2 cup diced bell pepper

- 1/4 cup diced red onion

- 1/4 cup chopped cilantro

- 2 tablespoons olive oil

- 2 tablespoons lime juice

- 1 teaspoon ground cumin

- Salt and pepper to taste

Instructions:

1. In a large bowl, combine black beans, corn kernels, diced bell pepper, diced red onion, and chopped cilantro.

2. In a small bowl, whisk together olive oil, lime juice, ground cumin, salt, and pepper.

3. Pour dressing over the salad and toss to coat evenly.

4. Serve chilled or at room temperature.

Servings: 2 **Nutritional Value per serving:** Calories: 250 | Protein: 10g | Carbohydrates: 35g | Fat: 8g | Fiber: 10g **Preparation Time:** 15 minutes

CHAPTER 5

1. Baked Lemon Herb Chicken

Ingredients:

- 2 boneless, skinless chicken breasts
- 2 tablespoons olive oil
- 2 cloves garlic, minced
- 1 tablespoon fresh lemon juice
- 1 teaspoon dried thyme
- 1 teaspoon dried rosemary
- Salt and pepper to taste

Instructions:

8. Preheat oven to 375°F (190°C).

9. In a small bowl, whisk together olive oil, minced garlic, lemon juice, dried thyme, dried rosemary, salt, and pepper.

10. Place chicken breasts in a baking dish and pour the olive oil mixture over them, ensuring they are evenly coated.

11. Bake for 25-30 minutes, or until chicken is cooked through and no longer pink in the center.

12.   Serve hot with your choice of sides.

Servings: 2 **Nutritional Value per serving:** Calories: 250 |
Protein: 30g | Carbohydrates: 2g | Fat: 12g | Fiber: 0g
Preparation Time: 35 minutes

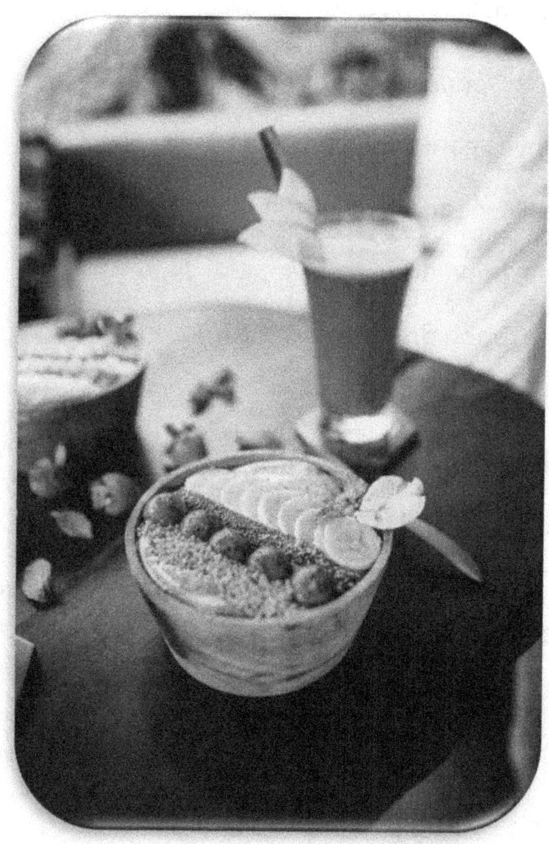

2. **Salmon and Asparagus Foil Packets**

Ingredients:

- 2 salmon fillets

- 1 bunch asparagus, trimmed

- 2 tablespoons olive oil

- 2 cloves garlic, minced

- 1 tablespoon lemon juice

- Salt and pepper to taste

Instructions:

6. Preheat oven to 400°F (200°C).

7. Cut two large pieces of aluminum foil and place a salmon fillet on each piece.

8. Divide the trimmed asparagus evenly between the two foil packets, placing it next to the salmon.

9. In a small bowl, whisk together olive oil, minced garlic, lemon juice, salt, and pepper.

10. Drizzle the olive oil mixture over the salmon and asparagus.

11. Fold the foil packets to seal them tightly.

12. Place the foil packets on a baking sheet and bake for 15-20 minutes, or until salmon is cooked through.

13. Carefully open the foil packets and serve hot.

Servings: 2 **Nutritional Value per serving:** Calories: 300 |
Protein: 30g | Carbohydrates: 5g | Fat: 18g | Fiber: 3g
Preparation Time: 25 minutes

3. **Vegetable Stir-Fry with Tofu**

Ingredients:

- 1 block firm tofu, drained and cubed
- 2 cups mixed vegetables (bell peppers, broccoli, carrots, snap peas)
- 2 cloves garlic, minced
- 2 tablespoons low-sodium soy sauce
- 1 tablespoon sesame oil
- 1 teaspoon grated ginger
- 1 tablespoon olive oil
- Salt and pepper to taste

Instructions:

0. Heat olive oil in a large skillet or wok over medium-high heat.

1. Add minced garlic and grated ginger to the skillet and cook for 1 minute.

2. Add cubed tofu to the skillet and cook until golden brown on all sides.

3. Add mixed vegetables to the skillet and stir-fry until tender-crisp.

4. In a small bowl, whisk together low-sodium soy sauce and sesame oil.

5. Pour the sauce over the tofu and vegetables in the skillet and toss to coat evenly.

6. Season with salt and pepper to taste.

7. Serve hot over cooked brown rice or quinoa.

Servings: 2 **Nutritional Value per serving:** Calories: 300 | Protein: 20g | Carbohydrates: 20g | Fat: 15g | Fiber: 6g
Preparation Time: 30 minutes

4. Spinach and Mushroom Stuffed Chicken Breast

Ingredients:

- 2 boneless, skinless chicken breasts
- 1 cup fresh spinach leaves
- 1/2 cup sliced mushrooms
- 1/4 cup diced onions
- 2 cloves garlic, minced
- 1/4 cup shredded low-fat mozzarella cheese
- 1 tablespoon olive oil
- Salt and pepper to taste

Instructions:

8. Preheat oven to 375°F (190°C).
9. In a skillet, heat olive oil over medium heat.
10. Add diced onions and minced garlic to the skillet and cook until softened.
11. Add sliced mushrooms and cook until they release their moisture.
12. Add fresh spinach leaves to the skillet and cook until wilted.
13. Remove from heat and let cool slightly.

14. Butterfly each chicken breast and season with salt and pepper.

15. Spoon the spinach and mushroom mixture onto one half of each chicken breast.

16. Sprinkle shredded mozzarella cheese over the spinach and mushrooms.

17. Fold the other half of each chicken breast over the filling to enclose it.

18. Secure with toothpicks if necessary.

19. Place stuffed chicken breasts in a baking dish and bake for 25-30 minutes, or until chicken is cooked through.

20. Serve hot with your choice of sides.

Servings: 2 **Nutritional Value per serving:** Calories: 300 | Protein: 35g | Carbohydrates: 5g | Fat: 15g | Fiber: 2g
Preparation Time: 45 minutes

5.   Turkey and Vegetable Skewers

Ingredients:

- 2 turkey breast cutlets, cut into cubes

- 1 zucchini, sliced

- 1 yellow squash, sliced

- 1 bell pepper, diced

- 1 red onion, diced

- 2 tablespoons olive oil

- 1 teaspoon dried oregano

- 1 teaspoon dried thyme

- Salt and pepper to taste

Instructions:

9. Preheat grill or grill pan to medium-high heat.

10. Thread turkey cubes and sliced vegetables onto skewers, alternating as desired.

11. In a small bowl, whisk together olive oil, dried oregano, dried thyme, salt, and pepper.

12. Brush the olive oil mixture over the turkey and vegetable skewers.

13. Grill skewers for 8-10 minutes, turning occasionally, until turkey is cooked through and vegetables are tender.

14. Serve hot with a side of whole grain rice or quinoa.

Servings: 2 **Nutritional Value per serving:** Calories: 280 | Protein: 30g | Carbohydrates: 15g | Fat: 12g | Fiber: 5g **Preparation Time:** 25 minutes

6. **Cauliflower Rice Stir-Fry with Shrimp**

Ingredients:

- 1 pound shrimp, peeled and deveined

- 4 cups cauliflower rice

- 1 cup mixed vegetables (bell peppers, broccoli, carrots, snap peas)

- 2 cloves garlic, minced

- 2 tablespoons low-sodium soy sauce

- 1 tablespoon sesame oil

- 1 tablespoon olive oil

- Salt and pepper to taste

Instructions:

8. Heat olive oil in a large skillet or wok over medium-high heat.

9. Add minced garlic to the skillet and cook for 1 minute.

10. Add shrimp to the skillet and cook until pink and opaque.

11. Remove shrimp from the skillet and set aside.

12. Add mixed vegetables to the skillet and stir-fry until tender-crisp.

13. Add cauliflower rice to the skillet and cook until heated through.

14. In a small bowl, whisk together low-sodium soy sauce and sesame oil.

15. Pour the sauce over the cauliflower rice and vegetables in the skillet.

16. Add cooked shrimp back to the skillet and toss to combine.

17. Season with salt and pepper to taste.

18. Serve hot.

Servings: 2 **Nutritional Value per serving:** Calories: 250 | Protein: 30g | Carbohydrates: 15g | Fat: 10g | Fiber: 5g **Preparation Time:** 20 minutes

7. **Vegetarian Chili**

Ingredients:

- 1 can (15 ounces) black beans, drained and rinsed
- 1 can (15 ounces) kidney beans, drained and rinsed
- 1 can (15 ounces) diced tomatoes
- 1 cup vegetable broth
- 1 onion, diced
- 2 cloves garlic, minced
- 1 bell pepper, diced
- 1 tablespoon olive oil
- 2 teaspoons chili powder
- 1 teaspoon ground cumin
- Salt and pepper to taste

Instructions:

11. Heat olive oil in a large pot over medium heat.

12. Add diced onion, minced garlic, and diced bell pepper to the pot and cook until softened.

13. Add chili powder and ground cumin to the

14. pot and cook for 1 minute, stirring constantly.

15. Add drained and rinsed black beans, kidney beans, diced tomatoes, and vegetable broth to the pot.

16. Bring the mixture to a boil, then reduce heat and simmer for 20-25 minutes, stirring occasionally.

17. Taste and adjust seasoning with salt and pepper if necessary.

18. Serve hot with a dollop of Greek yogurt or shredded cheese if desired.

Servings: 4 **Nutritional Value per serving:** Calories: 250 | Protein: 12g | Carbohydrates: 35g | Fat: 5g | Fiber: 12g **Preparation Time:** 30 minutes

8. **Baked Cod with Lemon Garlic Butter**

Ingredients:

- 2 cod fillets

- 2 tablespoons unsalted butter, melted

- 2 cloves garlic, minced

- 1 tablespoon fresh lemon juice

- 1 teaspoon lemon zest

- 1 teaspoon chopped fresh parsley

- Salt and pepper to taste

Instructions:

7. Preheat oven to 400°F (200°C).

8. Place cod fillets in a baking dish lined with parchment paper.

9. In a small bowl, whisk together melted butter, minced garlic, lemon juice, lemon zest, chopped parsley, salt, and pepper.

10. Pour the lemon garlic butter mixture over the cod fillets, ensuring they are evenly coated.

11. Bake for 15-20 minutes, or until fish is opaque and flakes easily with a fork.

12. Serve hot with steamed vegetables or a side salad.

Servings: 2 **Nutritional Value per serving:** Calories: 200 |
Protein: 20g | Carbohydrates: 2g | Fat: 12g | Fiber: 0g
Preparation Time: 25 minutes

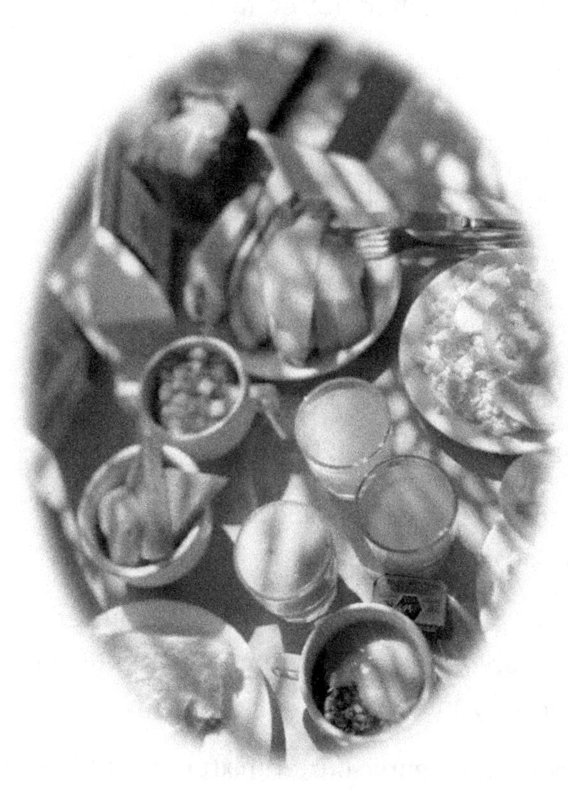

9. **Vegetable and Lentil Curry**

Ingredients:

- 1 cup dried green lentils, rinsed
- 2 cups vegetable broth
- 1 onion, diced
- 2 cloves garlic, minced
- 1 bell pepper, diced
- 1 zucchini, diced
- 1 cup diced tomatoes
- 1 can (13.5 ounces) coconut milk
- 2 tablespoons curry powder
- 1 tablespoon olive oil
- Salt and pepper to taste

Instructions:

11. In a large pot, heat olive oil over medium heat.

12. Add diced onion and minced garlic to the pot and cook until softened.

13. Add curry powder to the pot and cook for 1 minute, stirring constantly.

14. Add diced bell pepper, diced zucchini, diced tomatoes, rinsed lentils, and vegetable broth to the pot.

15. Bring the mixture to a boil, then reduce heat and simmer for 20-25 minutes, or until lentils are tender.

16. Stir in coconut milk and simmer for an additional 5 minutes.

17. Taste and adjust seasoning with salt and pepper if necessary.

18. Serve hot with cooked brown rice or quinoa.

Servings: 4 **Nutritional Value per serving:** Calories: 300 | Protein: 15g | Carbohydrates: 35g | Fat: 10g | Fiber: 12g **Preparation Time:** 40 minutes

10. Grilled Vegetable and Quinoa Salad

Ingredients:

- 1 cup cooked quinoa
- 1 zucchini, sliced
- 1 yellow squash, sliced
- 1 bell pepper, sliced
- 1 red onion, sliced
- 1 cup cherry tomatoes, halved
- 2 tablespoons balsamic vinegar
- 2 tablespoons olive oil
- 1 teaspoon Dijon mustard
- 1 teaspoon honey (optional)
- Salt and pepper to taste

Instructions:

1. Preheat grill to medium-high heat.
2. In a large bowl, toss sliced zucchini, yellow squash, bell pepper, and red onion with olive oil, salt, and pepper.
3. Grill vegetables for 5-7 minutes on each side, or until tender and lightly charred.

4. Remove vegetables from the grill and let cool slightly.

5. In a small bowl, whisk together balsamic vinegar, Dijon mustard, and honey (if using).

6. In a large bowl, combine cooked quinoa, grilled vegetables, halved cherry tomatoes, and balsamic vinaigrette.

7. Toss to coat evenly.

8. Serve warm or at room temperature.

Servings: 4 **Nutritional Value per serving:** Calories: 250 | Protein: 6g | Carbohydrates: 35g | Fat: 10g | Fiber: 6g
Preparation Time: 30 minutes

CONCLUSION

In conclusion, embracing a diet rich in osteoporosis-friendly juicing and smoothies offers not only a delicious culinary journey but also a profound opportunity to nurture your body and safeguard your skeletal health. These vibrant concoctions, brimming with essential nutrients like calcium, vitamin D, potassium, and magnesium, serve as potent elixirs for fortifying bones and combating the degenerative effects of osteoporosis.

By incorporating these rejuvenating beverages into your daily routine, you embark on a transformative path towards holistic well-being. With each sip, you nourish your body from within, replenishing it with the vital elements crucial for maintaining strong and resilient bones. Moreover, the anti-inflammatory properties of these ingredients work tirelessly to alleviate discomfort and enhance mobility, empowering you to lead a vibrant and active lifestyle well into your golden years.

Beyond the physical benefits, embracing this nutrient-dense diet represents a profound act of self-care and empowerment. It signifies a commitment to prioritizing your health and investing in a future filled with vitality and vitality. As you savor each sip of these revitalizing elixirs, you are not only nourishing your body but also nurturing your spirit, cultivating a deep sense of gratitude for the incredible vessel that carries you through life's journey.

Therefore, I urge you to embark on this flavorful adventure with an open heart and a steadfast determination to embrace the transformative power of nutrition. Together, let us raise our glasses to a future filled with strength, resilience, and boundless vitality. Cheers to your health and well-being!